Mediterrane Recipes for Beginners

The Complete Beginner's Guide,
Delicious Recipes to Get you Started with
Balanced Eating Plan

Healthy Kitchen

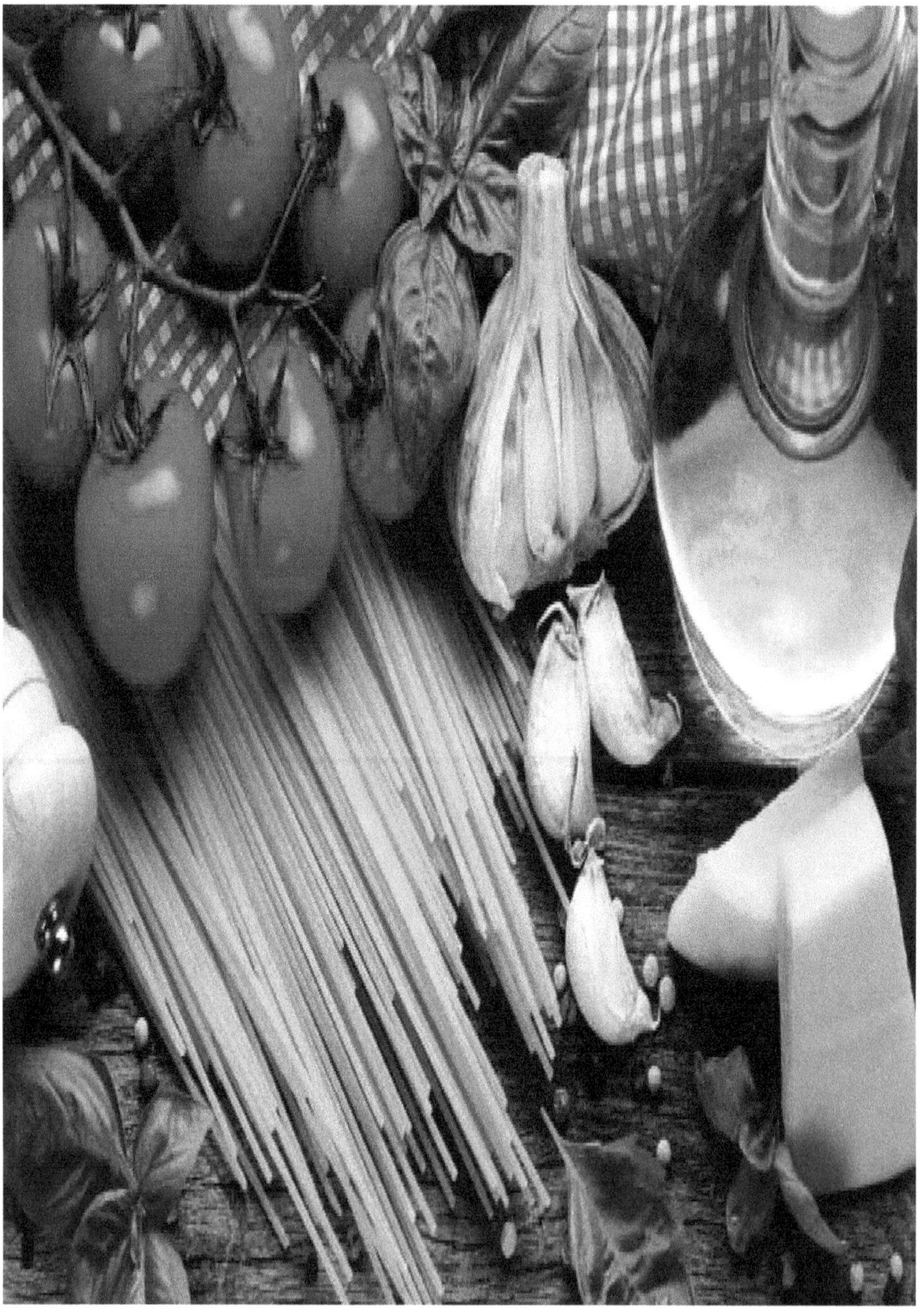

liable for any hardship or damages that may befall them after undertaking information described herein.

Additionally, the information in the following pages is intended only for informational purposes and should thus be thought of as universal. As befitting its nature, it is presented without assurance regarding its prolonged validity or interim quality. Trademarks that are mentioned are done without written consent and can in no way be considered an endorsement from the trademark holder.

Sommario

—
5

INTRODUCTION

The Mediterranean Diet's History

While this diet was first brought to light in 1945, until the 1990s, when people started to grow a newfound knowledge of what they were eating, it did not really reach mainstream levels. This is about the time when fitness programs started to surface on TV and healthy eating started to become popular again. The Mediterranean diet is based on the premise that there is a much lower risk of heart disease among people in these regions than in people with comparable fat consumption in other areas of the world. For instance, year after year, a person living in the United States and a person living in Greece might consume the exact same amount of fat, but the American would have a greater risk of suffering from heart disease because certain elements of his or her diet are missing.

Start your Diet

Stay Hydrated

Once you've started and are fully immersed in the Mediterranean diet, you might notice that you've started to feel a little bit weak, and a little bit colder, than you're used to.

The Mediterranean diet places an emphasis on trying to cut out as much sodium from your diet as possible, which is very healthy for some of us who already have high sodium levels. Sodium, obviously is found in salt, and so we proceed to cut out salt – and then drink enough water to drain every last drop of sodium from our bodies. When it comes to hydration, the biological mechanisms for keeping us saturated and quenched rely on an equal balance of sodium and potassium. Sodium can be found in your interstitial fluid, and potassium can be found inside our cytoplasm – two sides of one wall. When you drink tons of water, sweat a lot at the gym, or both, your sodium leaves your body in your urine and your sweat. Potassium, on the other hand, is only really lost through the urine – and even then, it's rare. This means that our bodies almost constantly need a refill on our sodium levels.

Vitamins and Supplements

Vitamins and minerals can be found in plants and animals, yes, but more often than not fruits and vegetables are much stronger sources. When consume another animal, we are consuming the sum total of all of the energy and nutrition that that animal has also consumed. This might sound like a sweet deal, but the pig you're eating used that energy in his own daily life, and therefore only has a tiny bit left to offer you. Plants, on the other hand, are first-hand sources of things like calcium, vitamin K, and vitamin C, which our bodies require daily doses of.

Meal Preparation and Portion Planning

If you haven't heard of the term "meal prep" before now, it's a beautiful day to learn something that will save you time, stress, and inches on your waistline. Meal prep, short for meal preparation, is a habit that was developed mostly by the body building community in order to accurately track your macronutrients. The basic idea behind meal prep is that each weekend, you manage your free time around cooking and preparing all of your meals for the upcoming week. While most meal preppers do their grocery shopping and cooking on Sundays, to keep their meals the freshest, you can choose to cook on a Saturday if that works better with your schedule. Meal prep each week uses one large grocery list of bulk ingredients to get all the supplies you need to make four dinners and four lunches of your choice. This means that you might have to do a bit of mental math quadrupling the serving size, but all you have to do is multiply each ingredient by four. Although you don't have to meal prep more than one meal with four portions each week, if you're already in the kitchen, you most likely have cooking time to work on something else.

Tracking Your Macronutrients

Wouldn't it be nice if you could have a full nutritional label for each of your home-cooked meals, just to make sure that your numbers are adding up in favor of weight loss? Oddly enough, tracking your macronutrients in order to calculate the nutritional value of each of your meals and portions is as easy as stepping on the scale. Not the scale in your bathroom, however. A food scale! If you've never had a good relationship with your weight and numbers, you might suddenly find that they aren't too bad after all. Food scales are used to measure, well, your food, but there's a slick system of online calculators and fitness applications for your smart phone that can take this number and turn it into magic. When you meal prep each week, keep track of your recipes diligently. Remember how you multiplied each of the ingredients on the list by four to create four servings? You're going to want to remember how much of each vegetable, fruit, grain, nut, and fat you cooked with. While you wait for your meal to finish cooking, find a large enough plastic container to fit all of your meals. Make sure it's clean and dry, and use the empty container to zero out your scale.

Counting Calories and Forming a Deficit

When it comes down to the technical science, there is one way and only one way to lose weight: by eating fewer calories in one day than your body requires to survive. Now, this doesn't mean that you can't lose weight for other reasons – be it water weight, as a result of stress, or simply working out harder. Although counting calories might not be the most fun way to lose weight, a calorie deficit is the only sure-fire way of guaranteeing that you reap all the weight loss benefits of the Mediterranean diet for your efforts. Scientifically, you already know that the healthy rate of weight loss for the average adult is between one and two pounds per week.

Get ready for a little bit more math, but it's nothing you can't handle in the name of a smaller waistline. One pound of fat equals around thirty-five hundred Calories, which means that your caloric deficit needs to account for that number, each week, without making too much of a dent on your regular nutrition. For most of us, we're used to eating between fifteen hundred and two thousand calories per day, which gives you a blessedly simply five hundred calorie deficit per day in order to reach your healthy weight loss goals. If you cut out exactly five hundred calories each day, you should be able to lose one pound of fat by the end of seven days. Granted, this estimate does take into account thirty minutes of daily exercise, but the results are still about the same when you rely on the scientific facts. If your age, height, weight, and sex predispose you to eat either more or less calories per day, you might want to consult with your doctor about the healthiest way for you to integrate a caloric deficit into your Mediterranean diet.

Goal Setting to Meet Your Achievements

On the subject of control, there are a few steps and activities that you should go through before you begin your Mediterranean diet just to make sure that you have clear and realistic goals in mind. Sitting down to set goals before embarking on a totally new diet routine will help you stay focused and committed during your Mediterranean diet. While a Mediterranean diet lifestyle certainly isn't as demanding as some of the crazy diet fads you see today, it can be a struggle to focus on eating natural fruits and vegetables that are more "salt of the Earth" foods than we're used to. You already know that when it comes to weight loss, you shouldn't expect to lose more than one to two pounds per week healthily while you're dieting. You are still welcome to set a weight loss goal with time in mind, but when it comes to the Mediterranean diet, you should set your goals for one month in the future.

Losing Weight

Further studies have provided examples of weight loss from the Mediterranean diet, as 322 individuals participated in an experiment where some individuals were exposed to a low-carb diet, others undertook a low-fat diet, and some consumed only a Mediterranean diet. The findings found that those on the Mediterranean diet had the greatest weight loss of all with 12 and 10 pounds respectively being lost by the top two participants. The study stressed that weight loss from the Mediterranean diet is successful and should be considered by anyone who has difficulty losing weight.

BREAKFAST

Healthy Scramble breakfast

Ingredients:

- 1 tsp. Extra virgin olive oil
- 4 green medium onions, chopped
- 1 tsp. Leaves of dried basil or 1 tbsp. New, chopped basil leaves
- 1 tomato medium, chopped
- Four eggs
- Pepper freshly ground

Directions:

1. Heat olive oil over medium heat in a medium nonstick skillet; sauté the green onions, stirring occasionally, for about 2 minutes.
2. Stir in the basil and tomatoes and cook, stirring periodically, for around 1 minute or until the tomatoes are fully cooked.
3. Beat the eggs thoroughly with a wire whisk or a fork in a small bowl and pour over the tomato mixture; cook for about 2 minutes.

4. Use the spatula to gently raise the cooked parts to allow the uncooked parts to flow to the bottom.

5. Continue to cook for about 3 minutes or until the eggs are completely cooked. Season and serve with pepper.

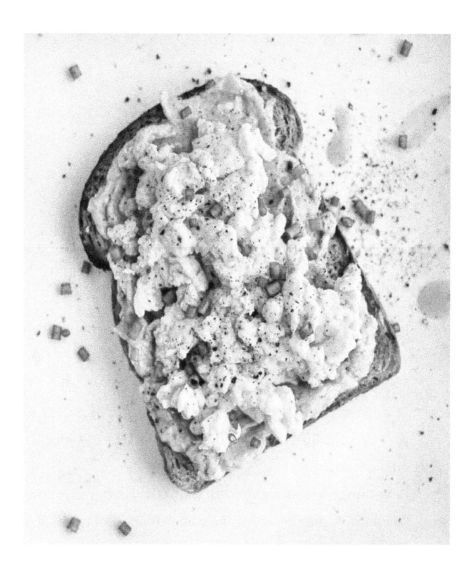

Avocado Egg Scramble

Ingredients:

- 4 eggs, beaten
- 1 white onion, diced
- 1 tablespoon avocado oil
- 1 avocado, finely chopped
- ½ teaspoon chili flakes
- 1 oz Cheddar cheese, shredded
- ½ teaspoon salt
- 1 tablespoon fresh parsley

Directions:

1. Pour avocado oil in the skillet and bring it to boil.
2. Then add diced onion and roast it until it is light brown.
3. Meanwhile, mix up together chili flakes, beaten eggs, and salt.
4. Pour the egg mixture over the cooked onion and cook the mixture for 1 minute over the medium heat.
5. After this, scramble the eggs well with the help of the fork or spatula. Cook the eggs until they are solid but soft.
6. After this, add chopped avocado and shredded cheese.
7. Stir the scramble well and transfer in the serving plates.
8. Sprinkle the meal with fresh parsley.

Garden Scramble

Ingredients:

- 1 teaspoon extra-virgin olive oil
- 1/2 cup diced yellow squash
- 1/2 cup diced green bell pepper
- 1/4 cup diced sweet white onion
- 6 cherry tomatoes, halved
- 1 tablespoon chopped fresh basil
- 1 tablespoon chopped fresh parsley
- 1/2 teaspoon salt
- 1/4 teaspoon freshly ground black pepper
- 8 large eggs, beaten

Directions:

1. In a large nonstick skillet, cook olive oil over medium heat. Add the squash, pepper, and onion and sauté for 4 minutes.
2. Add the tomatoes, basil, and parsley and season. Sauté for 1 minute, then pour the beaten eggs over the vegetables. Close and reduce the heat to low.
3. Cook for 6 minutes, making sure that the center is no longer runny.
4. To serve, slide the frittata onto a platter and cut into wedges.

Egg, Pancetta, and Spinach Benedict

Ingredients:

- 1/4 cup diced pancetta
- 2 cups baby spinach leaves
- 1/4 teaspoon freshly ground black pepper
- 1/4 teaspoon salt, or to taste
- 2 large eggs
- Extra-virgin olive oil (optional)
- 1 whole-grain English muffin, toasted

Directions:

1. In a medium, heavy skillet, brown the pancetta over medium-low heat for about 5 minutes, stirring frequently, until crisp on all sides.
2. Stir in the spinach, pepper, and salt if desired (it may not need any, depending on how salty the pancetta is). Cook, stirring occasionally, until the spinach is just wilted, about 5 minutes. Transfer the mixture to a medium bowl.
3. Crack the eggs into the same pan (add olive oil if the pan looks dry), and cook until the whites are just opaque, 3 to 4 minutes. Carefully flip the eggs and continue cooking for 30 seconds to 1 minute until done to your preferred degree for over-easy eggs.

4. Situate muffin half on each of 2 plates and top each with half of the spinach mixture and 1 egg, yolk side up. Pierce the yolks just before serving.

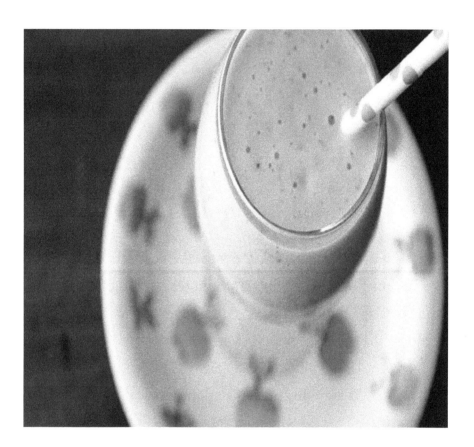

Peach Sunrise Smoothie

Ingredients:

- 1 large unpeeled peach, pitted and sliced (about 1/2 cup)
- 6 ounces vanilla or peach low-fat Greek yogurt
- 2 tablespoons low-fat milk
- 6 to 8 ice cubes

Directions:

Incorporate all ingredients in a blender and blend until thick and creamy. Serve immediately.

Oat and Fruit Parfait

Ingredients:

- 1/2 cup whole-grain rolled oats
- 1/2 cup walnut pieces
- 1 teaspoon honey
- 1 cup sliced fresh strawberries
- 11/2 cups (12 ounces) vanilla low-fat Greek yogurt
- Fresh mint leaves for garnish

Directions:

1. Preheat the oven to 300°F.
2. Spread the oats and walnuts in a single layer on a baking sheet.
3. Toast the oats and nuts just until you begin to smell the nuts, 10 to 12 minutes. Remove the pan from the oven and set aside.
4. In a small microwave-safe bowl, heat the honey just until warm, about 30 seconds. Add the strawberries and stir to coat.
5. Place 1 tablespoon of the strawberries in the bottom of each of 2 dessert dishes or 8-ounce glasses. Add a portion of yogurt and then a portion of oats and repeat the layers until the containers are full, ending with the berries. Serve immediately or chill until ready to eat.

Savory Avocado Spread

Ingredients:

- 1 ripe avocado
- 1 teaspoon lemon juice
- 6 boneless sardine filets
- 1/4 cup diced sweet white onion
- 1 stalk celery, diced
- 1/2 teaspoon salt
- 1/4 teaspoon black pepper

Directions:

1. In a blender, pulse avocado, lemon juice, and sardine filets
2. Spoon the mixture into a small bowl and add the onion, celery, salt, and pepper. Mix well with a fork and serve as desired.

Garlicky Broiled Sardines

Ingredients:

- 4 (3.25-ounce) cans sardines packed in water or olive oil
- 2 tablespoons extra-virgin olive oil
- 4 garlic cloves, minced
- 1/2 teaspoon red pepper flakes
- 1/2 teaspoon salt
- 1/4 teaspoon black pepper

Directions:

1. Preheat the broiler. Line a baking dish with aluminum foil. Lay sardines in a single layer on the foil.
2. Combine the olive oil (if using), garlic, and red pepper flakes in a small bowl and spoon over each sardine. Season with salt and pepper.
3. Broil just until sizzling, 2 to 3 minutes.
4. To serve, place 4 sardines on each plate and top with any remaining garlic mixture that has collected in the baking dish.

Almond Chia Porridge

Ingredients:

- 3 cups organic almond milk
- 1/3 cup chia seeds, dried
- 1 teaspoon vanilla extract
- 1 tablespoon honey
- ¼ teaspoon ground cardamom

Directions:

1. Pour almond milk in the saucepan and bring it to boil.
2. Then chill the almond milk to the room temperature (or appx. For 10-15 minutes).
3. Add vanilla extract, honey, and ground cardamom. Stir well.
4. After this, add chia seeds and stir again.
5. Close the lid and let chia seeds soak the liquid for 20-25 minutes.
6. Transfer the cooked porridge into the serving ramekins.

Cocoa Oatmeal

Ingredients:

- 1 ½ cup oatmeal
- 1 tablespoon cocoa powder
- ½ cup heavy cream
- ¼ cup of water
- 1 teaspoon vanilla extract
- 1 tablespoon butter
- 2 tablespoons Splenda

Directions:

1. Mix up together oatmeal with cocoa powder and Splenda.
2. Transfer the mixture in the saucepan.
3. Add vanilla extract, water, and heavy cream. Stir it gently with the help of the spatula.
4. Close the lid and cook it for 10-15 minutes over the medium-low heat.
5. Remove the cooked cocoa oatmeal from the heat and add butter. Stir it well.

Avocado Milk Shake

Ingredients:

- 1 avocado, peeled, pitted
- 2 tablespoons of liquid honey
- ½ teaspoon vanilla extract
- ½ cup heavy cream
- 1 cup milk
- 1/3 cup ice cubes

Directions:

1. Chop the avocado and put in the food processor.
2. Add liquid honey, vanilla extract, heavy cream, milk, and ice cubes.
3. Blend the mixture until it smooth.
4. Pour the cooked milkshake in the serving glasses.

Coconut Clam Chowder

Ingredients:

- 6 oz clams, chopped
- 1 cup heavy cream
- 1/4 onion, sliced
- 1 cup celery, chopped
- 1 lb cauliflower, chopped
- 1 cup fish broth
- 1 bay leaf
- 2 cups of coconut milk
- Salt

Directions:

1. Add all ingredients except clams and heavy cream and stir well.
2. Seal pot with lid and cook on high for 5 minutes.
3. Once done, release pressure using quick release. Remove lid.
4. Add heavy cream and clams and stir well and cook on sauté mode for 2 minutes.
5. Stir well and serve.

MAIN DISH RECIPES

Spanish Paella Saffron Rice, Seafood, And Chicken

Ingredients:

- Twelve Medium Shrimps
- 7 clams that are hard-shelled
- 1⁄2 pound garlic-seasoned sausage of smoked pork
- 2 pounds of skinless, boneless chicken, sliced into freshly ground pepper dash bits.
- 3⁄4 teaspoon of salt from garlic
- 1⁄2 cup of olive oil extra virgin
- 1⁄4 pound of slightly boneless pork, cut into 1⁄2-inch cubes
- 1⁄2 cup of onion chopped
- 1⁄2 medium red, seeded and sliced bell pepper
- 1⁄2 yellow medium bell pepper, seeded and sliced
- 1 big, peeled and finely chopped tomato
- 2 cloves of fresh, crushed garlic
- Long-grain rice 3 cups
- 1⁄2 teaspoon of salt
- 1⁄4 teaspoon of ground saffron with 6 cups of water

- 1 cup frozen peas, thoroughly defrosted

Directions:

1. Steam shrimp until only pink in a tiny amount of water, then set aside. Scrub the clams under running water, then steam to coat them with just enough water.

2. Remove from the water with a slotted spoon when the clams open, and set aside. In many places, prick sausage with a fork, put in a heavy skillet, and cover with cold water. Bring water to a boil and heat to a low level.

3. Let the sausages cook, uncovered, for 15 minutes. Drain the sausages well, slice and set aside into 1/4-inch round bits. Rinse the chicken, pat dry, and apply the pepper and garlic salt to the seasoning.

4. Heat 1/4 cup of olive oil in a large skillet, add the chicken bits, and fry until golden brown. Take the browned chicken out of the skillet and put it on a paper towel lined tray.

5. Add the bits of sausage to the pan, brown them quickly and then drain them on a plate lined with paper towels. Remove the olive oil from the skillet and use paper towels to dry the skillet.

6. Heat 1/4 cup of fresh olive oil in the same skillet, until sweet. Attach cubes of pork and easily brown. Add the onions, red and yellow bell peppers, garlic, and tomatoes.

7. Cook the vegetables and meat until tender, stirring constantly. Only set aside. Put the rice, salt, saffron, and 6

cups of water into a large pot; bring to a boil and cover, stirring occasionally, until the rice is tender. In an oven-safe casserole dish, move the rice, shrimp and remaining liquid, clams, bacon, chicken and pork cubes, and vegetables.

8. Sprinkle the peas over the mixture, put the pan on a 400-degree oven bottom rack, and bake for 25-30 minutes or until the liquid is absorbed. You don't stir. Remove from the oven when the paella is baked, cover with clean kitchen towels, and let stand for 5 minutes. Immediately serve. Note: Oven should be preheated 30 minutes before the paella is located inside.

Balsamic Beef

Ingredients:

- 2 pounds boneless chuck roast
- 1 tablespoon olive oil

  Rub
- 1 teaspoon garlic powder
- ½ teaspoon onion powder
- 1 teaspoon sea salt
- ½ teaspoon black pepper

  Sauce
- ½ cup balsamic vinegar
- 2 tablespoons honey
- 1 tablespoon honey mustard
- 1 cup beef broth
- 1 tablespoon tapioca

Directions:

1. Incorporate all of the ingredients for the rub.
2. In a separate bowl, mix the balsamic vinegar, honey, honey mustard, and beef broth.
3. Coat the roast in olive oil, then rub in the spices from the rub mix.
4. Place the roast in the slow cooker and then pour the sauce over the top.

5. Select slow cooker to low and cook for 8 hours.

6. If you want to thicken, pour the liquid into a saucepan and heat to boiling on the stovetop. Stir in the flour until smooth and let simmer until the sauce thickens.

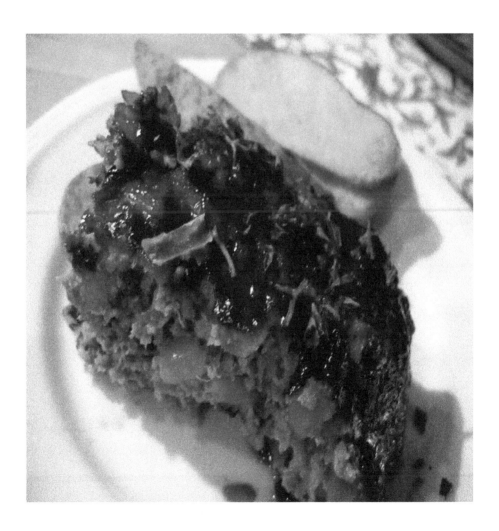

Veal Pot Roast

Ingredients:

- 2 tablespoons olive oil
- Salt and pepper
- 3-pound boneless veal roast
- 4 medium carrots, peeled
- 2 parsnips, peeled and halved
- 2 white turnips, peeled and quartered
- 10 garlic cloves, peeled
- 2 sprigs fresh thyme
- 1 orange, scrubbed and zested
- 1 cup chicken or veal stock

Directions:

1. Heat a large skillet over medium-high heat.
2. Coat veal roast all over with olive oil, then season with salt and pepper.
3. When the skillet is hot, add the veal roast and sear on all sides.
4. Once roast is cooked on all sides, transfer it to the slow cooker.
   5. Toss the carrots, parsnips, turnips, and garlic into the skillet. Stir and cook for about 5 minutes—not all the

way through, just to get some of the brown bits from the veal and give them a bit of color.

6. Transfer the vegetables to the slow cooker, placing them all around the meat.

7. Top the roast with the thyme and the zest from the orange. Slice

8. orange in half and squeeze the juice over the top of the meat.

9. Add the chicken stock, then cook the roast on low for 5 hours.

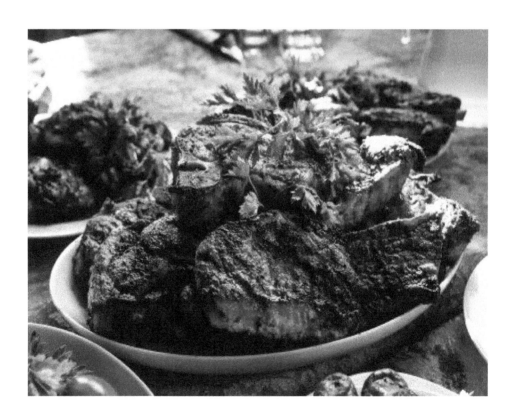

Mediterranean Rice and Sausage

Ingredients:

- 1½ pounds Italian sausage, crumbled
- 1 medium onion, chopped
- 2 tablespoons steak sauce
- 2 cups long grain rice, uncooked
- 1 (14-ounce) can diced tomatoes with juice ½ cup water
- 1 medium green pepper, diced

Directions:

1. Spray your slow cooker with olive oil or nonstick cooking spray.
2. Add the sausage, onion, and steak sauce to the slow cooker.
3. Cook on low for 8 to 10 hours.
4. After 8 hours, add the rice, tomatoes, water and green pepper. Stir to combine thoroughly.
5. Cook for 20 to 25 minutes.

Spanish Meatballs

Ingredients:

- 1-pound ground turkey
- 1-pound ground pork
- 2 eggs
- 1 (20-ounce) can diced tomatoes
- ¾ cup sweet onion, minced, divided
- ¼ cup plus 1 tablespoon breadcrumbs
- 3 tablespoons fresh parsley, chopped
- 1½ teaspoons cumin
- 1½ teaspoons paprika (sweet or hot)

Directions:

1. Spray the slow cooker with olive oil.
2. In a mixing bowl, mix ground meat, eggs, about half of the onions, the breadcrumbs, and the spices.
3. Wash your hands and mix together until everything is well combined. Shape into meatballs.
4. Mix 2 tablespoons of olive oil over medium heat. When the skillet and oil are hot, add the meatballs and brown on all sides. When they are done, transfer them to the slow cooker.

5. Add the rest of the onions and the tomatoes to the skillet and allow them to cook for a few minutes, scraping the brown bits from the meatballs up to add flavor.

6. Pour the tomatoes over the meatballs in the slow cooker and cook on low for 5 hours.

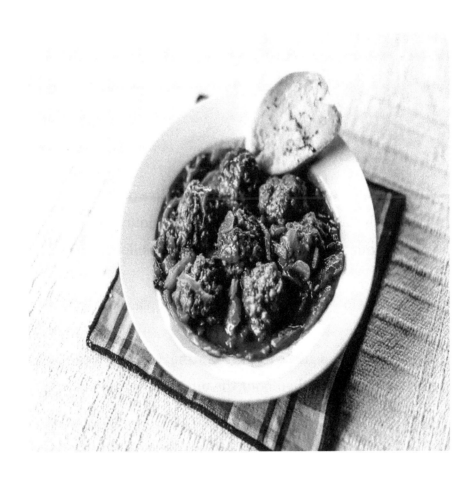

Lamb Shanks with Red Wine

Ingredients:

- 2 tablespoons olive oil
- 2 tablespoons flour
- 4 lamb shanks, trimmed
- 1 onion, chopped
- 2 garlic cloves, crushed
- 2/3 cup red wine
- 3 cups tomato sauce

Directions:

1. Heat a skillet over high heat. Add the olive oil.
2. Season the lamb shanks then roll in the flour. Shake off excess flour and place the shanks in the skillet to brown on all sides.
3. Spray the slow cooker with olive oil and place the browned shanks in the slow cooker.
4. Add the crushed garlic to the red wine. Mix with the tomato sauce and then pour the mixture over the lamb shanks and cook on low for 5– 6 hours

Leg of Lamb with Rosemary and Garlic

Ingredients:

- 3–4-pound leg of lamb
- 4 garlic cloves, sliced thin
- 5–8 sprigs fresh rosemary (more if desired)
- 2 tablespoons olive oil
- 1 lemon, halved
- ¼ cup flour

Directions:

1. Put skillet over high heat and pour olive oil.
2. When the olive oil is hot, add the leg of lamb and sear on both sides until brown.
3. Spray the slow cooker with olive oil and then transfer the lamb to the slow cooker.
4. Squeeze the lemon over the meat and then place in the pot next to the lamb.
5. Take a sharp knife and make small incisions in the meat, then stuff the holes you created with rosemary and garlic.
6. Place any remaining rosemary and garlic on top of the roast.
7. Cook on low for 8 hours.

Lemon Honey Lamb Shoulder

Ingredients:

- 3 cloves garlic, thinly sliced
- 1 tablespoon fresh rosemary, chopped
- 1 teaspoon lemon zest, grated
- ½ teaspoon each salt and pepper
- 4–5-pound boneless lamb shoulder roast
- 3 tablespoons lemon juice
- 1 tablespoon honey
- 6 shallots, quartered
- 2 teaspoons cornstarch

Directions:

1. Stir garlic, rosemary, lemon zest, salt, and pepper.
2. Rub the spice mixture into the lamb shoulder. Make sure to coat the whole roast.
3. Spray the slow cooker with olive oil and add the lamb.
4. Mix together the honey and lemon juice and then pour over the meat.
5. Arrange the shallots beside the meat in the slow cooker.
6. Cook on low for 8 hours.
7. Serve. You can make a gravy by transferring the juice from the slow cooker to a medium saucepan. Thoroughly mix the cornstarch into a little water until smooth. Then mix into e

juice and bring to a simmer. Simmer until mixture thickens.

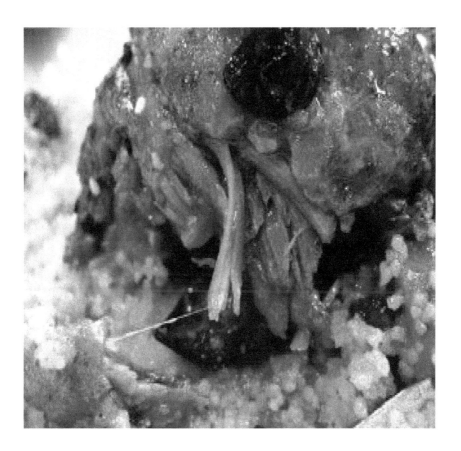

Italian Shredded Pork Stew

Ingredients:

- 2 medium sweet potatoes
- 2 cups fresh kale, chopped
- 1 large onion, chopped
- 4 cloves garlic, minced
- 1 2½–3½ pound boneless pork shoulder butt roast
- 1 (14-ounce) can cannellini beans
- 1½ teaspoons Italian seasoning
- ½ teaspoon salt
- ½ teaspoon pepper
- 3 (14½-ounce) cans chicken broth
- Sour cream (optional)

Directions:

1. Coat slow cooker with nonstick cooking spray or olive oil.
2. Place the cubed sweet potatoes, kale, garlic and onion into the slow cooker.
3. Add the pork shoulder on top of the potatoes.
4. Add the beans, Italian seasoning salt, and pepper.
5. Pour the chicken broth over the meat.
6. Cook on low for 8 hours.
7. Serve with sour cream, if desired.

Parmesan Honey Pork Loin Roast

Ingredients:

- 3-pound pork loin
- 2/3 cup grated parmesan cheese
- ½ cup honey
- 3 tablespoons soy sauce
- 1 tablespoon oregano
- 1 tablespoon basil
- 2 tablespoons garlic, chopped
- 2 tablespoons olive oil
- ½ teaspoon salt
- 2 tablespoons cornstarch
- ¼ cup chicken broth

Directions:

1. Spray your slow cooker with olive oil or nonstick cooking spray.
2. Place the pork loin in the slow cooker.
3. In a small mixing bowl, combine the cheese, honey, soy sauce, oregano, basil, garlic, olive oil, and salt. Stir with a fork to combine well, then pour over the pork loin.
4. Cook in low for 5–6 hours.
5. Remove the pork loin and put on a serving platter.

6. Pour the juices from the slow cooker into a small saucepan.
7. Create a slurry by mixing the cornstarch into the chicken broth and whisking until smooth.
8. Bring the contents of the saucepan to a boil, then whisk in the slurry and let simmer until thickened. Pour over the pork loin and serve.

Steamed Sea Bass

Ingredients:

- Sea bass (or grouper) for 2 pounds,
- 1-inch-thick whole fillets,
- 2 1/2 tablespoons extra virgin olive oil if possible,
- 8 thin red onion slices
- 2 cloves of fresh, thinly sliced garlic
- 10 sprigs of medium fresh dill
- 8 slices of lemon, 1/2-inch thick
- 1 tablespoon of rinsed and drained capers,
- The taste of freshly ground pepper
- 2 tablespoons of dry white sea salt wine, to taste

Directions:

1. Cut the parchment paper and put it on a baking sheet twice the size of the fish. Place the fish on paper and drizzle it with olive oil. On top of the trout, scatter the onion slices, garlic, dill sprigs, and lemon slices.

2. Sprinkle with freshly ground pepper and a splash of wine by adding capers. Wrap parchment paper around fish to create a seal so that steam does not escape during baking, folding top and tucking ends under fish.

3. Bake in the oven for 30 minutes at 400 degrees. Check for thickness after 20 minutes; the fish in the middle should

be opaque. Rewrap tightly if not, and finish baking for an extra 10 minutes.

4. Place the fish, still wrapped in parchment, on a platter for serving. When ready to eat, open parchment; sprinkle on salt and serve instantly.

5. This dish goes well with rice, steamed and/or couscous vegetables.

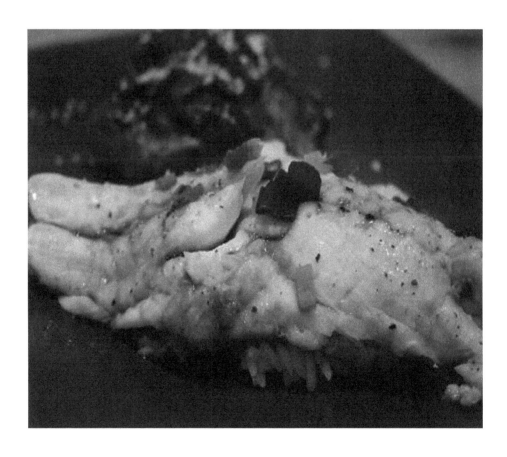

Spicy Chicken with Couscous

Ingredients:

- ¼ teaspoon cumin field
- ¼ teaspoon turmeric from the field
- 1 teaspoon cayenne ground
- 1 pound skinless, boneless chicken breasts, cut into 1-inch strips
- 1 tablespoon of extra-virgin olive oil
- 5 cloves of fresh, finely minced garlic

- Low-sodium, fat-free chicken broth,
- 1 (16-ounce) can 1 cup of peas new
- 1 big white, diced onion
- 1 red bell pepper medium, diced
- Salt and to taste, freshly ground pepper
- 1 Cup Couscous
- ¼ cup of fresh cilantro chopped, for garnish

Directions:

1. Combine the cumin, turmeric, and cayenne and spray the chicken evenly. Strips, set aside then. Heat olive oil in a nonstick skillet over medium-high heat, until hot. Add the chicken and garlic and cook until the chicken is lightly browned for around 3 minutes.

2. In the skillet, add broth, peas, onion, red bell pepper, and salt and pepper to taste; bring to a boil, reduce heat and simmer for 2-3 minutes until chicken is cooked through. Incorporate the couscous, cover, and remove from the sun. Let it stand until it absorbs liquid. Cilantro garnish.

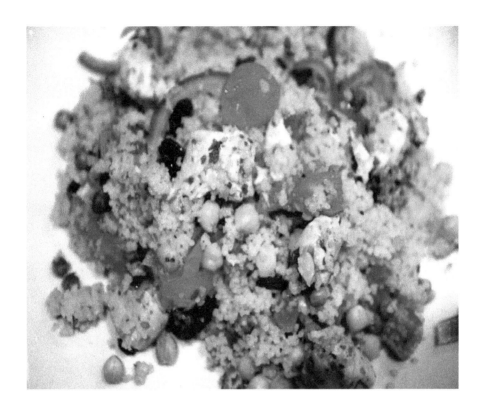

Citrus Scallops and Shrimp

Ingredients:

- 3 cloves of fresh, finely minced garlic
- 2½ tablespoons of olive oil extra virgin, split
- 1½ pounds of arugula new
- Half a pound of broad sea scallops, cut in half
- 12 big, peeled and deveined shrimps
- 4 ounces of fresh juice of oranges
- ½ Pink Grapefruit Juice
- The Juice of 1 Lime
- The Juice of 1 Lemon
- 1 honey teaspoon
- ½ teaspoon of fine orange zest shredded
- ½ teaspoon of lime zest, finely shredded
- Salt and to taste, freshly ground pepper
- 2 scallions, thinly sliced for garnish

Directions:

1. Sauté garlic in 1 tablespoon olive oil for 1 minute in a large skillet over medium-high heat; do not brown. Add the arugula, cover and cook until the greens are wilted, for 1 minute. Heat the remaining olive oil in a separate skillet over a medium-high heat.

2. Add the scallops and shrimp and cook until the scallops and shrimp are opaque and pink, turning gently to avoid burning. Move the scallops and shrimp to a heated plate, cover and set aside to keep warm.
3. Reserve the skillet and set it aside with seafood drippings. Mix the orange juice, grapefruit juice, lime juice, sugar, lemon juice, orange and lime zest together.
4. Pour the mixture of juice into a reserved skillet of seafood and return the skillet to medium heat. To loosen any browned bits, swirl the bottom and sides of the pan and mix them into the juices.
5. Bring it to a boil and cook until the volume of liquid is reduced to half. Add salt and pepper to taste, cook and remove from the heat for a couple of seconds. Drain and divide wilted arugula between 4 plates, middle placed.
6. Divide the shrimp and scallops into 4 sections and place them on top of the arugula. Glaze the juice over the seafood and sprinkle with the scallions.

Italian Poached Scallops

Ingredients:

- 1 cup of fresh juice from oranges
- New sea scallops for 1 pound
- 2 teaspoons of orange peel grated
- 1 tiny ripe tomato with plum, chopped
- 1 teaspoon new chopped marjoram
- 2 teaspoons of sour cream low-fat
- Salt and to taste, freshly ground pepper

Directions:

1. Bring the orange juice to a boil in a big, nonstick skillet over medium heat. Lower the heat and add the orange peel and scallops.

2. Cover and boil for five minutes or until the scallops are soft and opaque. Remove from heat and pass scallops to a plate; cover to stay warm.

3. To the orange juice sauce, add the tomato and marjoram and simmer for around 2 minutes until the liquid reduces to half the original amount. Add the sour cream and cook until the sauce is thick.

4. To taste, apply salt and pepper. Put the scallops back in the skillet, mix with the sauce, and heat up. Serve with risotto and/or vegetables right away.

Light Breaded Grilled Grouper

Ingredients:

- ½ cup of pitted mature Kalamata olives
- ¼ cup of simple crumbs for bread
- 1 tablespoon of rinsed and drained capers,
- 1 extra virgin olive oil teaspoon
- 1 lemon juice teaspoon
- 1 new garlic clove
- 4 (4-ounce) fillet groupers
- For garnish, 4-8 lime wedges

Directions:

1. Heat the high-heat grill; put the oil-rubbed fish-grilling pan on the grill rack to heat up. Process the olives, breadcrumbs, capers, olive oil, lemon juice, and garlic in a food processor until smooth.
2. Brush the olive oil mixture on each side of the fillets and put the fillets on the hot grill pan. Grill the fillets for 5 minutes, uncovered.
3. Brush with the olive oil mixture before turning the fillets over then turn and grill for 5 more minutes or until the fillets flake easily. Take the fillets out of the grill, put them on a dish and serve immediately, garnished with lime wedges.
4. This recipe suits well with couscous or seasoned rice.

Black Olives and Lamb

Ingredients:

- Extra virgin olive oil for 2 tablespoons
- 3 cloves of fresh, crushed garlic
- 1–2 new parsley sprigs
- 2 pounds lean lamb field
- 2 tomatoes, chopped and peeled
- ½ teaspoon of rosemary dried
- 12 black olives pitted, halved
- 1 cup of white dry wine

Directions:

1. In a large skillet, heat olive oil; add garlic and parsley and sauté until golden brown.
2. Add the lamb, continue cooking and stir frequently until the lamb is browned. Stir in the onions, rosemary, wine, and olives.
3. Stir, cover, and cook for 5 minutes or until the lamb is cooked and most of the liquid has evaporated. With rice, serve.

Blackened Swordfish

Ingredients:

- Olive oil for 2 tablespoons
- 1 tablespoon of lemon juice that has been freshly squeezed
- 4 (6-ounce) steaks for swordfish
- 1 tablespoon of option Creole seasoning mix, divided
- Wedges with lemon

Directions:

1. In a 450-degree oven, preheat a cast-iron skillet. In a small dish, combine the olive oil and the lemon juice. Dip each steak in lemon mixture to coat and season with 1/4 tablespoon Creole seasoning on both sides of each steak. Place the steaks in a preheated skillet and cook for 2 minutes or so.
2. Switch over the steaks and proceed to cook until blackens and fish flakes are
3. seasoned quickly. Don't make steaks burn. Remove the steaks from the heat and serve with lemon wedges right away.

Roasted Pork Florentine

Ingredients:

- 4 pounds of lean pork loin
- 4 cloves new garlic, sliced thin
- 1/2 teaspoon of rosemary dried
- Four cloves of fresh garlic, whole garlic
- Water 5–6 tablespoons
- 6 to 8 tablespoons of hearty red wine (do not use wine to cook) Salt and to taste, freshly ground pepper

Directions:

1. If the loin skin has not already been graded, cut lines about 1/8 inch apart into the skin. On one hand, cut through the flesh into the bone and insert the garlic slices and the rosemary.
2. In a 350-degree oven with water and wine, press all the garlic cloves into the scored loin skin and put the loin into a roasting pan.
3. Sprinkle salt and pepper on the loin generously and roast for 2-2½ hours or until the meat is very tender but still moist, basting periodically. Serve with your favorite vegetables, with a choice.

Chicken with Pomegranate Sauce

Ingredients:

- 4 pounds of skinless chicken breast, boneless, cut into small pieces
- 2 tsp. of paprika
- Salt and to taste, freshly ground pepper
- 1/4 cup of olive oil extra virgin
- Four cloves of fresh, minced garlic
- 2 yellow medium onions, chopped
- 1/4 cup of fresh parsley chopped
- 1 tiny, finely chopped hot banana pepper
- 3 tablespoons of Thick Molasses of Pomegranate
- 3-4 cups of frozen, undrained, chunky tomatoes

Directions:

1. Wash the chicken and remove the fat, then cut it into small bits. Sprinkle with salt and pepper and paprika. In a saucepan, heat the olive oil, add the chicken bits, and fry for around 2-3 minutes.
2. For another 2-3 minutes, add garlic and stir-fry. Add the onions, parsley, spicy banana pepper, thick molasses of pomegranate, and liquid tomatoes; cover and bring to a boil. Cook for about 30 minutes over medium-low heat, until the chicken is tender. With rice, serve.

Braised Duck with Fennel Root

Ingredients:

- 1/4 cup olive oil
- 1 whole duck, cleaned
- 3 teaspoon fresh rosemary
- 2 garlic cloves, minced
- 3 fennel bulbs, cut into chunks
- 1/2 cup sherry

Directions:

1. Preheat the oven to 375 degrees.
2. Cook olive oil in a Dutch oven.
3. Season the duck, including the cavity, with the rosemary, garlic, sea salt, and freshly ground pepper.
4. Place the duck in the oil, and cook it for 10–15 minutes, turning as necessary to brown all sides.
5. Add the fennel bulbs and cook an additional 5 minutes.
6. Pour the sherry over the duck and fennel, cover and cook in the oven for 30–45 minutes, or until internal temperature of the duck is 140–150 degrees at its thickest part.
7. Allow duck to sit for 15 minutes before serving.

Turkey Burgers with Mango Salsa

Ingredients:

- 1½ pounds ground turkey breast
- 1 teaspoon sea salt, divided
- ¼ teaspoon freshly ground black pepper
- 2 tablespoons extra-virgin olive oil
- 2 mangos, peeled, pitted, and cubed
- ½ red onion, finely chopped
- Juice of 1 lime
- 1 garlic clove, minced
- ½ jalapeño pepper, seeded and finely minced
- 2 tablespoons chopped fresh cilantro leaves

Directions:

1. Form the turkey breast into 4 patties and season with ½ teaspoon of sea salt and the pepper.
2. In a nonstick skillet over medium-high heat, heat the olive oil until it shimmers.
3. Add the turkey patties and cook for about 5 minutes per side until browned.
4. While the patties cook, mix together the mango, red onion, lime juice, garlic, jalapeño, cilantro, and remaining ½ teaspoon of sea salt in a small bowl. Spoon the salsa over the turkey patties and serve.

Herb-Roasted Turkey Breast

Ingredients:

- 2 tablespoons extra-virgin olive oil
- 4 garlic cloves, minced
- Zest of 1 lemon
- 1 tablespoon fresh thyme leaves
- 1 tablespoon fresh rosemary leaves
- 2 tablespoons fresh Italian parsley leaves
- 1 teaspoon ground mustard
- 1 teaspoon sea salt
- ¼ teaspoon black pepper
- 1 (6-pound) bone-in, skin-on turkey breast
- 1 cup dry white wine

Directions:

1. Preheat the oven to 325°F.
2. Scourge olive oil, garlic, lemon zest, thyme, rosemary, parsley, mustard, sea salt, and pepper. Lay out herb mixture evenly over the surface of the turkey breast, and loosen the skin and rub underneath as well. Place the turkey breast in a roasting pan on a rack, skin-side up.
3. Pour the wine in the pan. Roast for 1 to 1½ hour. Take out from the oven and rest for 20 minutes, tented with aluminum foil to keep it warm, before carving.

Chicken Sausage and Peppers

Ingredients:

- 2 tablespoons extra-virgin olive oil
- 6 Italian chicken sausage links
- 1 onion
- 1 red bell pepper
- 1 green bell pepper
- 3 garlic cloves, minced
- ½ cup dry white wine
- ½ teaspoon sea salt
- ¼ teaspoon freshly ground black pepper
- Pinch red pepper flakes

Directions:

1. In a skillet at medium-high heat, cook olive oil.
2. Add the sausages and cook for 5 to 7 minutes, turning occasionally, until browned, and they reach an internal temperature of 165°F. With tongs, remove the sausage from the pan and set aside on a platter, tented with aluminum foil to keep warm.
3. Put skillet back to the heat and add the onion, red bell pepper, and green bell pepper. Cook for 5 to 7 minutes.
4. Cook garlic 30 seconds, stirring constantly.

5. Stir in the wine, sea salt, pepper, and red pepper flakes. Scrape and fold in any browned bits from the bottom. Simmer for about 4 minutes more. Spoon the peppers over the sausages and serve.

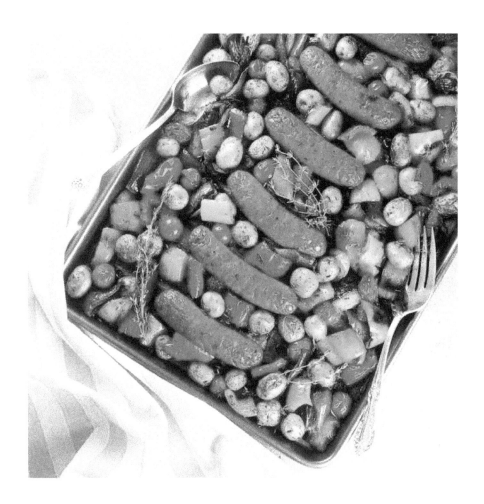

Chicken Piccata

Ingredients:

- ½ cup whole-wheat flour
- ½ teaspoon sea salt
- 1/8 teaspoon freshly ground black pepper
- 1½ pounds boneless
- 3 tablespoons extra-virgin olive oil
- 1 cup unsalted chicken broth
- ½ cup dry white wine
- Juice of 1 lemon
- Zest of 1 lemon
- ¼ cup capers, drained and rinsed
- ¼ cup chopped fresh parsley leaves

Directions:

1. In a shallow dish, whisk the flour, sea salt, and pepper. Dredge the chicken in the flour and tap off any excess.
2. In a pan over medium-high heat, cook olive oil.
3. Add the chicken and cook for about 4 minutes. Remove the chicken from the pan and set aside, tented with aluminum foil to keep warm.
4. Return back to the heat and mix broth, wine, lemon juice, and lemon zest, and capers. Simmer for 3 to 4 minutes, stirring. Remove the skillet from the heat and return the hicken to the pan. Turn to coat. Stir in the parsley and serve.

One-Pan Tuscan Chicken

Ingredients:

- ¼ cup extra-virgin olive oil, divided
- 1-pound boneless chicken
- 1 onion
- 1 red bell pepper
- 3 garlic cloves
- ½ cup dry white wine
- 2 (14-ounce) can tomatoes
- 1 (14-ounce) can white beans
- 1 tablespoon dried Italian seasoning
- ½ teaspoon sea salt
- 1/8 teaspoon freshly ground black pepper
- 1/8 teaspoon red pepper flakes
- ¼ cup chopped fresh basil leaves

Directions:

1. In a huge skillet over medium-high heat, preheat 2 tablespoons of olive oil.
2. Add the chicken and cook for about 6 minutes, stirring. Take out the chicken and set aside on a platter, tented with aluminum foil to keep warm.
3. Return the skillet to the heat and heat the remaining 2 tablespoons of olive oil.

4. Add the onion and red bell pepper. Cook for about 5 minutes.
5. Cook garlic for 30 seconds.
6. Stir in the wine. Cook for 1 minute, stirring.
7. Add the crushed and chopped tomatoes, white beans, Italian seasoning, sea salt, pepper, and red pepper flakes. Bring to a simmer and reduce the heat to medium. Cook for 5 minutes, stirring occasionally.
8. Take chicken and any juices that have collected back to the skillet. Cook for 1 to 2 minutes. Pull out from the heat and stir in the basil before serving.

Chicken Kapama

Ingredients:

- 1 (32-ounce) can chopped tomatoes
- ¼ cup dry white wine
- 2 tablespoons tomato paste
- 3 tablespoons extra-virgin olive oil
- ¼ teaspoon red pepper flakes
- 1 teaspoon ground allspice
- ½ teaspoon dried oregano
- 2 whole cloves
- 1 cinnamon stick
- ½ teaspoon sea salt
- 1/8 teaspoon black pepper
- 4 boneless, skinless chicken breast halves

Directions:

1. In pot over medium-high heat, mix the tomatoes, wine, tomato paste, olive oil, red pepper flakes, allspice, oregano, cloves, cinnamon stick, sea salt, and pepper. Bring to a simmer, stirring occasionally.

2. Adjust heat to medium-low and simmer for 30 minutes, stirring occasionally. Remove and discard the whole cloves and cinnamon stick from the sauce and let the sauce cool.

3. Preheat the oven to 350°F.

4. Situate chicken in a 9-by-13-inch baking dish. Drizzle sauce over the chicken and cover the pan with aluminum foil. Bake for 45 minutes.

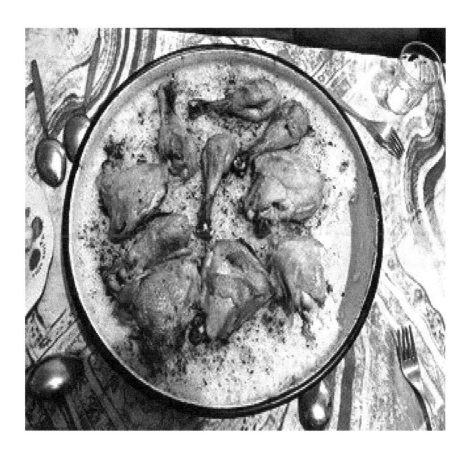

Spinach and Feta–Stuffed Chicken Breasts

Ingredients:

- 2 tablespoons extra-virgin olive oil
- 1-pound fresh baby spinach
- 3 garlic cloves, minced
- Zest of 1 lemon
- ½ teaspoon sea salt
- 1/8 teaspoon freshly ground black pepper
- ½ cup crumbled feta cheese
- 4 chicken breast halves

Dircctions:

1. Preheat the oven to 350°F.
2. Preheat oil and skillet over medium-high heat
3. Cook spinach for 3 to 4 minutes.
4. Cook garlic, lemon zest, sea salt, and pepper. Cool slightly and mix in the cheese.
5. Spread the spinach and cheese mixture in an even layer over the chicken pieces and roll the breast around the filling. Hold closed with toothpicks or butcher's twine.
6. Place the breasts in a 9-by-13-inch baking dish and bake for 30 to 40 minutes. Take away from the oven and let rest for 5 minutes before slicing and serving.

Rosemary Baked Chicken Drumsticks

Ingredients:

- 2 tablespoons chopped fresh rosemary leaves
- 1 teaspoon garlic powder
- ½ teaspoon sea salt
- 1/8 teaspoon freshly ground black pepper
- Zest of 1 lemon
- 12 chicken drumsticks

Directions:

1. Preheat the oven to 350°F.
2. Blend rosemary, garlic powder, sea salt, pepper, and lemon zest.
3. Situate drumsticks in a 9-by-13-inch baking dish and sprinkle with the rosemary mixture. Bake for about 1 hour.

Chicken with Onions, Potatoes, Figs, and Carrots

Ingredients:

- 2 cups fingerling potatoes, halved
- 4 fresh figs, quartered
- 2 carrots, julienned
- 2 tablespoons extra-virgin olive oil
- 1 teaspoon sea salt, divided
- ¼ teaspoon freshly ground black pepper
- 4 chicken leg-thigh quarters
- 2 tablespoons chopped fresh parsley leaves

Directions:

1. Preheat the oven to 425°F.
2. In a small bowl, toss the potatoes, figs, and carrots with the olive oil, ½ teaspoon of sea salt, and the pepper. Spread in a 9-by-13-inch baking dish.
3. Rub chicken with the remaining ½ teaspoon of sea salt. Place it on top of the vegetables. Bake for 35 to 45 minutes.
4. Sprinkle with the parsley and serve.

SEAFOOD RECIPES

Baked Bean Fish Meal

Ingredients:

- 1 tablespoon balsamic vinegar

- 2 ½ cups green beans

- 1-pint cherry or grape tomatoes

- 4 (4-ounce each) fish fillets, such as cod or tilapia

- 2 tablespoons olive oil

Directions:

1. Preheat an oven to 400 degrees. Grease two baking sheets with some olive oil or olive oil spray. Arrange 2 fish fillets on each sheet. In a mixing bowl, pour olive oil and vinegar. Combine to mix well with each other.

2. Mix green beans and tomatoes. Combine to mix well with each other. Combine both mixtures well with each other. Add mixture equally over fish fillets. Bake for 6-8 minutes, until fish opaque and easy to flake. Serve warm.

Tuna Nutty Salad

Ingredients:

- 1 tablespoon chopped tarragon
- 1 stalk celery, trimmed and finely diced
- 1 medium shallot, diced
- 3 tablespoons chopped chives
- 1 (5-ounce) can tuna (covered in olive oil)
- 1 teaspoon Dijon mustard
- 2-3 tablespoons mayonnaise
- 1/4 teaspoon salt
- 1/8 teaspoon pepper
- 1/4 cup pine nuts, toasted

Directions:

1. In a large salad bowl, add tuna, shallot, chives, tarragon, and celery. Combine to mix well with each other. In a mixing bowl, add mayonnaise, mustard, salt, and black pepper.

2. Combine to mix well with each other. Add mayonnaise mixture to salad bowl; toss well to combine. Add pine nuts and toss again. Serve fresh.

Creamy Shrimp Soup

Ingredients:

- 1-pound medium shrimp

- 1 leek, both whites and light green parts, sliced

- 1 medium fennel bulb, chopped

- 2 tablespoons olive oil

- 3 stalks celery, chopped

- 1 clove garlic, minced

- Sea salt and ground pepper to taste

- 4 cups vegetable or chicken broth

- 1 tablespoon fennel seeds

- 2 tablespoons light cream

- Juice of 1 lemon

Directions:

1. Take a medium-large cooking pot or Dutch oven, heat oil over medium heat. Add celery, leek, and fennel and stir-cook for about 15 minutes, until vegetables are softened and browned. Add garlic; season with black pepper and sea salt to taste. Add fennel seed and stir.

2. Pour broth and bring to a boil. Over low heat, simmer mixture for about 20 minutes, stir in between. Add shrimp and cook until just pink for 3 minutes. Mix in cream and lemon juice; serve warm.

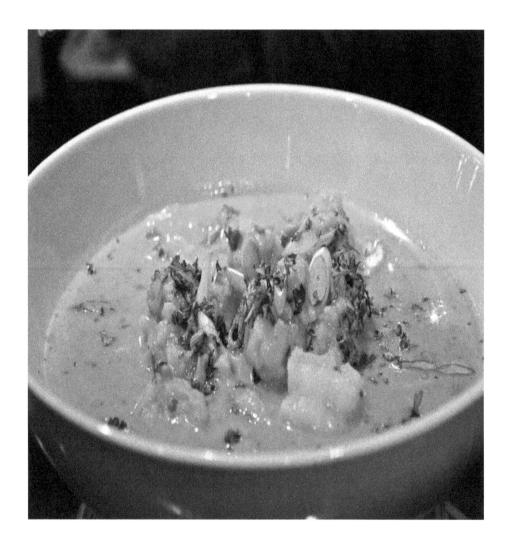

Spiced Salmon with Vegetable Quinoa
Ingredients:

- 1 cup uncooked quinoa

- 1 teaspoon of salt, divided in half

- ¾ cup cucumbers, seeds removed, diced

- 1 cup of cherry tomatoes, halved

- ¼ cup red onion, minced

- 4 fresh basil leaves, cut in thin slices

- Zest from one lemon

- ¼ teaspoon black pepper

- 1 teaspoon cumin

- ½ teaspoon paprika

- 4 (5-oz.) salmon fillets

- 8 lemon wedges

- ¼ cup fresh parsley, chopped

Directions:

1. To a medium-sized saucepan, add the quinoa, 2 cups of water, and ½ teaspoons of the salt. Heat these until the water is boiling, then lower the temperature until it is simmering. Cover the pan and let it cook 20 minutes or as long as the quinoa package instructs. Turn off the burner under the quinoa and allow it to sit, covered, for at least another 5 minutes before serving.

2. Right before serving, add the onion, tomatoes, cucumbers, basil leaves, and lemon zest to the quinoa and use a spoon to stir everything together gently. In the meantime (while the quinoa cooks), prepare the salmon. Turn on the oven broiler to high and make sure a rack is in the lower part of the oven. To a small bowl, add the following components: black pepper, ½ teaspoon of the salt, cumin, and paprika. Stir them together.

3. Place foil over the top of a glass or aluminum baking sheet, then spray it with nonstick cooking spray. Place salmon fillets on the foil. Rub the spice mixture over each fillet (about ½ teaspoons of the spice mixture per fillet). Add the lemon wedges to the pan edges near the salmon.

4. Cook the salmon under the broiler for 8-10 minutes. Your goal is for the salmon to flake apart easily with a fork. Sprinkle the salmon with the parsley, then serve it with the lemon wedges and vegetable parsley. Enjoy!

Mushroom Cod Stew

Ingredients:

- 2 tablespoons extra-virgin olive oil

- 2 garlic cloves, minced

- 1 can tomato

- 2 cups chopped onion

- ¾ teaspoon smoked paprika

- a (12-ounce) jar roasted red peppers

- 1/3 cup dry red wine

- ¼ teaspoon kosher or sea salt

- ¼ teaspoon black pepper

- 1 cup black olives

- 1 ½ pounds cod fillets, cut into 1-inch pieces

- 3 cups sliced mushrooms

Directions:

1. Get medium-large cooking pot, warm up oil over medium heat. Add onions and stir-cook for 4 minutes.

2. Add garlic and smoked paprika; cook for 1 minute, stirring often. Add tomatoes with juice, roasted peppers, olives, wine, pepper, and salt; stir gently.

3. Boil mixture. Add the cod and mushrooms; turn down heat to medium. Close and cook until the cod is easy to flake, stir in between. Serve warm.

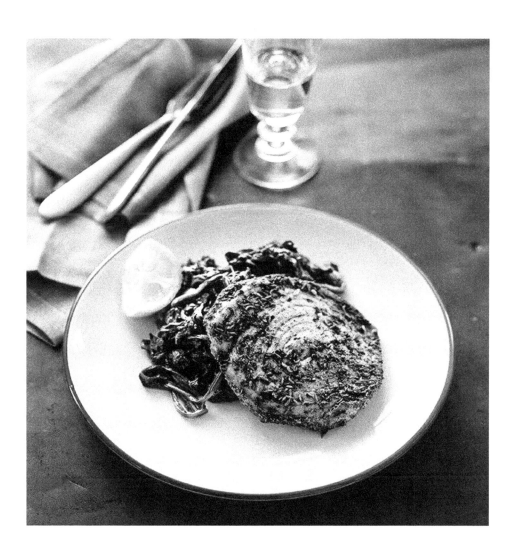

Spiced Swordfish

Ingredients:

- 4 (7 ounces each) swordfish steaks

- 1/2 teaspoon ground black pepper

- 12 cloves of garlic, peeled

- 3/4 teaspoon salt

- 1 1/2 teaspoon ground cumin

- 1 teaspoon paprika

- 1 teaspoon coriander

- 3 tablespoons lemon juice

- 1/3 cup olive oil

Directions:

1. Take a blender or food processor, open the lid and add all the ingredients except for swordfish. Close the lid and blend to make a smooth mixture. Pat dry fish steaks; coat evenly with the prepared spice mixture.

2. Add them over an aluminum foil, cover and refrigerator for 1 hour. Preheat a griddle pan over high heat, pour oil and heat it. Add fish steaks; stir-cook for 5-6 minutes per side until cooked through and evenly browned. Serve warm.

Orange Fish Meal

Ingredients:

- ¼ teaspoon kosher or sea salt

- 1 tablespoon extra-virgin olive oil

- 1 tablespoon orange juice

- 4 (4-ounce) tilapia fillets, with or without skin

- ¼ cup chopped red onion

- 1 avocado, pitted, skinned, and sliced

Directions:

1. Take a baking dish of 9-inch; add olive oil, orange juice, and salt. Combine well. Add fish fillets and coat well.

2. Add onions over fish fillets. Cover with a plastic wrap. Microwave for 3 minutes until fish is cooked well and easy to flake. Serve warm with sliced avocado on top.

Baked Cod with Vegetables

Ingredients:

- 1 pound (454 g) thick cod fillet, cut into 4 even portions
- ¼ teaspoon onion powder (optional)
- ¼ teaspoon paprika
- 3 tablespoons extra-virgin olive oil
- 4 medium scallions
- ½ cup fresh chopped basil, divided
- 3 tablespoons minced garlic (optional)
- 2 teaspoons salt
- 2 teaspoons freshly ground black pepper
- ¼ teaspoon dry marjoram (optional)
- 6 sun-dried tomato slices
- ½ cup dry white wine
- ½ cup crumbled feta cheese
- 1 (15-ounce / 425-g) can oil-packed artichoke hearts, drained
- 1 lemon, sliced

- 1 cup pitted kalamata olives

- 1 teaspoon capers (optional)

- 4 small red potatoes, quartered

Directions:

1. Set oven to 375°F (190°C).

2. Season the fish with paprika and onion powder (if desired).

3. Heat an ovenproof skillet over medium heat and sear the top side of the cod for about 1 minute until golden. Set aside.

4. Heat the olive oil in the same skillet over medium heat. Add the scallions, ¼ cup of basil, garlic (if desired), salt, pepper, marjoram (if desired), tomato slices, and white wine and stir to combine. Boil then removes from heat.

5. Evenly spread the sauce on the bottom of skillet. Place the cod on top of the tomato basil sauce and scatter with feta cheese. Place the artichokes in the skillet and top with the lemon slices.

6. Scatter with the olives, capers (if desired), and the remaining ¼ cup of basil. Pullout from the heat and transfer to the preheated oven. Bake for 15 to 20 minutes

7. Meanwhile, place the quartered potatoes on a baking sheet or wrapped in aluminum foil. Bake in the oven for 15 minutes.

8. Cool for 5 minutes before serving.

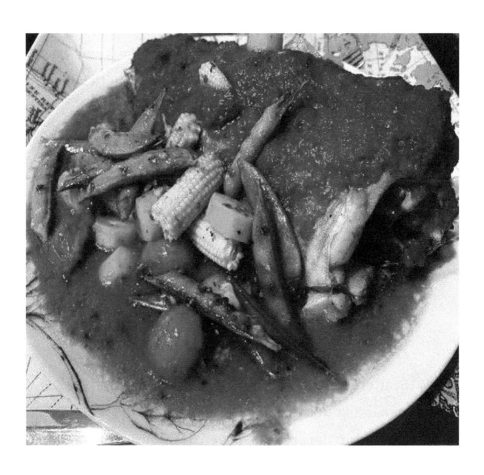

Slow Cooker Salmon in Foil

Ingredients:

- 2 (6-ounce / 170-g) salmon fillets
- 1 tablespoon olive oil
- 2 cloves garlic, minced
- ½ tablespoon lime juice
- 1 teaspoon finely chopped fresh parsley
- ¼ teaspoon black pepper

Directions:

1. Spread a length of foil onto a work surface and place the salmon fillets in the middle.

2. Blend olive oil, garlic, lime juice, parsley, and black pepper. Brush the mixture over the fillets. Fold the foil over and crimp the sides to make a packet.

3. Place the packet into the slow cooker, cover, and cook on High for 2 hours

4. Serve hot.

Dill Chutney Salmon

Ingredients:

Chutney:

- ¼ cup fresh dill

- ¼ cup extra virgin olive oil

- Juice from ½ lemon

- Sea salt, to taste

Fish:

- 2 cups water

- 2 salmon fillets

- Juice from ½ lemon

- ¼ teaspoon paprika

- Salt and freshly ground pepper to taste

Directions:

1. Pulse all the chutney ingredients in a food processor until creamy. Set aside.

2. Add the water and steamer basket to the Instant Pot. Place salmon fillets, skin-side down, on the steamer basket. Drizzle the lemon juice over salmon and sprinkle with the paprika.

3. Secure the lid. Select the Manual mode and set the cooking time for 3 minutes at High Pressure.

4. Once cooking is complete, do a quick pressure release. Carefully open the lid.

5. Season the fillets with pepper and salt to taste. Serve topped with the dill chutney.

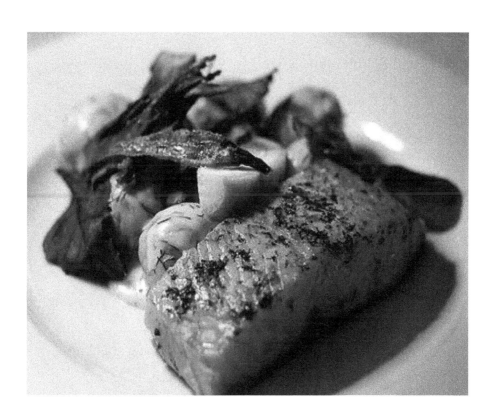

Garlic-Butter Parmesan Salmon and Asparagus

Ingredients:

- 2 (6-ounce / 170-g) salmon fillets, skin on and patted dry

- Pink Himalayan salt

- Freshly ground black pepper, to taste

- 1 pound (454 g) fresh asparagus, ends snapped off

- 3 tablespoons almond butter

- 2 garlic cloves, minced

- ¼ cup grated Parmesan cheese

Directions:

1. Prep oven to 400°F (205°C). Line a baking sheet with aluminum foil.

2. Season both sides of the salmon fillets.

3. Situate salmon in the middle of the baking sheet and arrange the asparagus around the salmon.

4. Heat the almond butter in a small saucepan over medium heat.

5. Cook minced garlic

6. Drizzle the garlic-butter sauce over the salmon and asparagus and scatter the Parmesan cheese on top.

7. Bake in the preheated oven for about 12 minutes. You can switch the oven to broil at the end of cooking time for about 3 minutes to get a nice char on the asparagus.

8. Let cool for 5 minutes before serving.

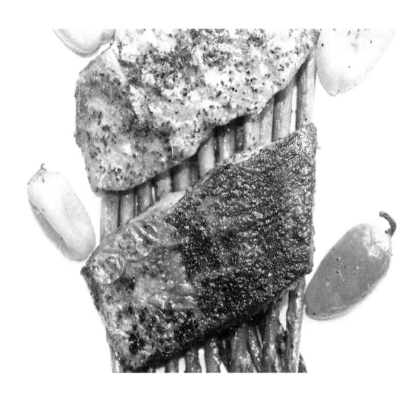

Lemon Rosemary Roasted Branzino

Ingredients:

- 4 tablespoons extra-virgin olive oil, divided
- 2 (8-ounce) Branzino fillets
- 1 garlic clove, minced
- 1 bunch scallions
- 10 to 12 small cherry tomatoes, halved
- 1 large carrot, cut into ¼-inch rounds
- ½ cup dry white wine
- 2 tablespoons paprika
- 2 teaspoons kosher salt
- ½ tablespoon ground chili pepper
- 2 rosemary sprigs or 1 tablespoon dried rosemary
- 1 small lemon, thinly sliced
- ½ cup sliced pitted kalamata olives

Direction:

1. Heat a large ovenproof skillet over high heat until hot, about 2 minutes. Add 1 tablespoon of olive oil and heat

2. Add the Branzino fillets, skin-side up, and sear for 2 minutes. Flip the fillets and cook. Set aside.

---

3. Swirl 2 tablespoons of olive oil around the skillet to coat evenly.

4. Add the garlic, scallions, tomatoes, and carrot, and sauté for 5 minutes

5. Add the wine, stirring until all ingredients are well combined. Carefully place the fish over the sauce.

6. Preheat the oven to 450°F (235°C).

7. Brush the fillets with the remaining 1 tablespoon of olive oil and season with paprika, salt, and chili pepper. Top each fillet with a rosemary sprig and lemon slices. Scatter the olives over fish and around the skillet.

8. Roast for about 10 minutes until the lemon slices are browned. Serve hot.

Grilled Lemon Pesto Salmon

Ingredients:

- 10 ounces (283 g) salmon fillet
- 2 tablespoons prepared pesto sauce
- 1 large fresh lemon, sliced
- Cooking spray

Directions:

1. Preheat the grill to medium-high heat. Spray the grill grates with cooking spray.

2. Season the salmon well. Spread the pesto sauce on top.

3. Make a bed of fresh lemon slices about the same size as the salmon fillet on the hot grill, and place the salmon on top of the lemon slices. Put any additional lemon slices on top of the salmon.

4. Grill the salmon for 10 minutes.

5. Serve hot.

Steamed Trout with Lemon Herb Crust

Ingredients:

- 3 tablespoons olive oil
- 3 garlic cloves, chopped
- 2 tablespoons fresh lemon juice
- 1 tablespoon chopped fresh mint
- 1 tablespoon chopped fresh parsley
- ¼ teaspoon dried ground thyme
- 1 teaspoon sea salt
- 1 pound (454 g) fresh trout (2 pieces)
- 2 cups fish stock

Directions:

1. Blend olive oil, garlic, lemon juice, mint, parsley, thyme, and salt. Brush the marinade onto the fish.

2. Insert a trivet in the Instant Pot. Fill in the fish stock and place the fish on the trivet.

3. Secure the lid. Select the Steam mode and set the cooking time for 15 minutes at High Pressure.

4. Once cooking is complete, do a quick pressure release. Carefully open the lid. Serve warm.

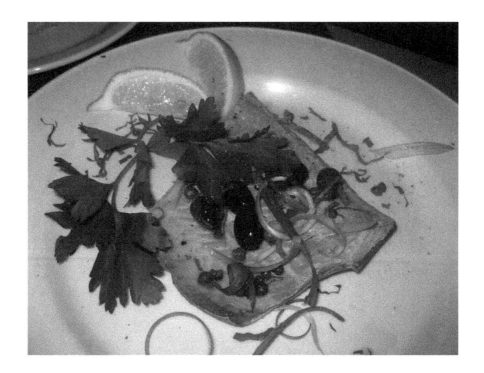

Roasted Trout Stuffed with Veggies

Ingredients:

- 2 (8-ounce) whole trout fillets
- 1 tablespoon extra-virgin olive oil
- ¼ teaspoon salt
- 1/8 teaspoon black pepper
- 1 small onion, thinly sliced
- ½ red bell pepper
- 1 poblano pepper
- 2 or 3 shiitake mushrooms, sliced
- 1 lemon, sliced

Directions:

1. Set oven to 425°F (220°C). Coat baking sheet with nonstick cooking spray.

2. Rub both trout fillets, inside and out, with the olive oil. Season with salt and pepper.

3. Mix together the onion, bell pepper, poblano pepper, and mushrooms in a large bowl. Stuff half of this mix into the cavity of each fillet. Top the mixture with 2 or 3 lemon slices inside each fillet.

4. Place the fish on the prepared baking sheet side by side. Roast in the preheated oven for 25 minutes

5. Pullout from the oven and serve on a plate.

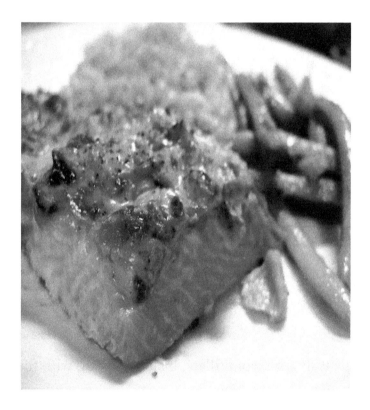

Lemony Trout with Caramelized Shallots

Ingredients:

Shallots:

- 1 teaspoon almond butter

- 2 shallots, thinly sliced

- Dash salt

Trout:

- 1 tablespoon almond butter

- 2 (4-ounce / 113-g) trout fillets

- 3 tablespoons capers

- ¼ cup freshly squeezed lemon juice

- ¼ teaspoon salt

- Dash freshly ground black pepper

- 1 lemon, thinly sliced

Directions:

For Shallots

1. Situate skillet over medium heat, cook the butter, shallots, and salt for 20 minutes, stirring every 5 minutes.

For Trout

2. Meanwhile, in another large skillet over medium heat, heat 1 teaspoon of almond butter.

3. Add the trout fillets and cook each side for 3 minutes, or until flaky. Transfer to a plate and set aside.

4. In the skillet used for the trout, stir in the capers, lemon juice, salt, and pepper, then bring to a simmer. Whisk in the remaining 1 tablespoon of almond butter. Spoon the sauce over the fish.

5. Garnish the fish with the lemon slices and caramelized shallots before serving.

Easy Tomato Tuna Melts

Ingredients:

- 1 (5-oz) can chunk light tuna packed in water

- 2 tablespoons plain Greek yogurt

- 2 tablespoons finely chopped celery

- 1 tablespoon finely chopped red onion

- 2 teaspoons freshly squeezed lemon juice

- 1 large tomato, cut into ¾-inch-thick rounds

- ½ cup shredded Cheddar cheese

Directions:

1. Preheat the broiler to High.

2. Stir together the tuna, yogurt, celery, red onion, lemon juice, and cayenne pepper in a medium bowl.

3. Place the tomato rounds on a baking sheet. Top each with some tuna salad and Cheddar cheese.

4. Broil for 3 to 4 minutes until the cheese is melted and bubbly. Cool for 5 minutes before serving.

Mackerel and Green Bean Salad

Ingredients:

- 2 cups green beans
- 1 tablespoon avocado oil
- 2 mackerel fillets
- 4 cups mixed salad greens
- 2 hard-boiled eggs, sliced
- 1 avocado, sliced
- 2 tablespoons lemon juice
- 2 tablespoons olive oil
- 1 teaspoon Dijon mustard
- Salt and black pepper, to taste

Directions:

1. Cook the green beans in pot of boiling water for about 3 minutes. Drain and set aside.

2. Melt the avocado oil in a pan over medium heat. Add the mackerel fillets and cook each side for 4 minutes.

3. Divide the greens between two salad bowls. Top with the mackerel, sliced egg, and avocado slices.

4. Scourge lemon juice, olive oil, mustard, salt, and pepper, and drizzle over the salad. Add the cooked green beans and toss to combine, then serve.

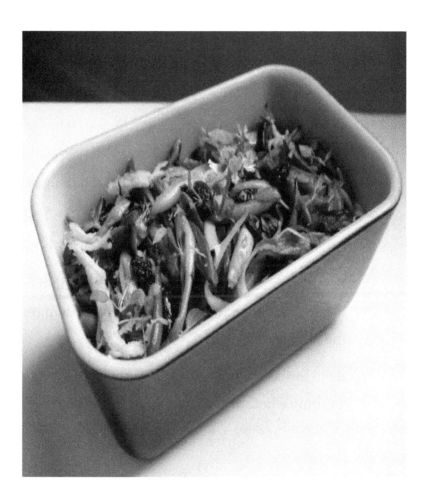

Hazelnut Crusted Sea Bass

Ingredients:

- 2 tablespoons almond butter

- 2 sea bass fillets

- 1/3 cup roasted hazelnuts

- A pinch of cayenne pepper

Directions:

1. Ready oven to 425°F (220°C). Line a baking dish with waxed paper.

2. Brush the almond butter over the fillets.

3. Pulse the hazelnuts and cayenne in a food processor. Coat the sea bass with the hazelnut mixture, then transfer to the baking dish.

4. Bake in the preheated oven for about 15 minutes. Cool for 5 minutes before serving.

Shrimp Zoodles

Ingredients:

- 2 tablespoons chopped parsley

- 2 teaspoons minced garlic

- 1 teaspoon salt

- ½ teaspoon black pepper

- 2 medium zucchinis, spiralized

- 3/4 pounds medium shrimp, peeled & deveined

- 1 tablespoon olive oil

- 1 lemon, juiced and zested

Directions:

1. Take a medium saucepan or skillet, add oil, lemon juice, lemon zest. Heat over medium heat. Add shrimps and stir-cook 1 minute per side.

2. Sauté garlic and red pepper flakes for 1 more minute. Add Zoodles and stir gently; cook for 3 minutes until cooked to satisfaction. Season well, serve warm with parsley on top.

Asparagus Trout Meal

Ingredients:

- 2 pounds trout fillets

- 1-pound asparagus

- 1 tablespoon olive oil

- 1 garlic clove, finely minced

- 1 scallion, thinly sliced

- 4 medium golden potatoes

- 2 Roma tomatoes, chopped

- 8 pitted kalamata olives, chopped

- 1 large carrot, thinly sliced

- 2 tablespoons dried parsley

- ¼ cup ground cumin

- 2 tablespoons paprika

- 1 tablespoon vegetable bouillon seasoning

- ½ cup dry white wine

Directions:

1. In a mixing bowl, add fish fillets, white pepper and salt. Combine to mix well with each other. Take a medium saucepan or skillet, add oil.

2. Heat over medium heat. Add asparagus, potatoes, garlic, white part scallion, and stir-cook until become softened for 4-5 minutes. Add tomatoes, carrot and olives; stir-cook for 6-7 minutes until turn tender. Add cumin, paprika, parsley, bouillon seasoning, and salt. Stir mixture well.

3. Mix in white wine and fish fillets. Over low heat, cover and simmer mixture for about 6 minutes until fish is easy to flake, stir in between. Serve warm with green scallions on top.

Kale Olive Tuna

Ingredients:

- 1 cup chopped onion

- 3 garlic cloves, minced

- 1 (2.25-ounce) can sliced olives

- 1-pound kale, chopped

- 3 tablespoons extra-virgin olive oil

- ¼ cup capers

- ¼ teaspoon crushed red pepper

- 2 teaspoons sugar

- 1 (15-ounce) can cannellini beans

- 2 (6-ounce) cans tuna in olive oil, un-drained

- ¼ teaspoon black pepper

- ¼ teaspoon kosher or sea salt

Directions:

1. Soak kale in boiling water for 2 minutes; drain and set aside. Take a medium-large cooking pot or stock pot, heat oil over medium heat.

2. Add onion and stir-cook until become translucent and softened. Add garlic and stir-cook until become fragrant for 1 minute.

3. Add olives, capers, and red pepper, and stir-cook for 1 minute. Mix in cooked kale and sugar. Over low heat, cover and simmer mixture for about 8-10 minutes, stir in between.

4. Add tuna, beans, pepper, and salt. Stir well and serve warm.

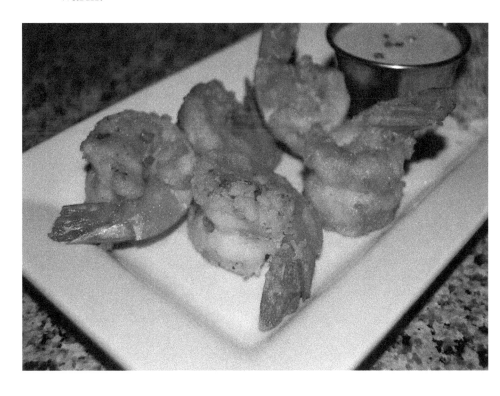

Tangy Rosemary Shrimps

Ingredients:

- 1 large orange, zested and peeled

- 3 garlic cloves, minced

- 1 ½ pounds raw shrimp, shells and tails removed

- 3 tablespoons olive oil

- 1 tablespoon chopped thyme

- 1 tablespoon chopped rosemary

- ¼ teaspoon black pepper

- ¼ teaspoon kosher or sea salt

Directions:

1.   Take a zip-top plastic bag, add orange zest, shrimps, 2 tablespoons olive oil, garlic, thyme, rosemary, salt, and black pepper. Shake well and set aside to marinate for 5 minutes.

2.   Take a medium saucepan or skillet, add 1 tablespoon olive oil. Heat over medium heat. Add shrimps and stir-cook for 2-3 minutes per side until totally pink and opaque.

3.   Slice orange into bite-sized wedges and add in a serving plate. Add shrimps and combine well. Serve fresh.

Asparagus Salmon

Ingredients:

- 8.8-ounce bunch asparagus

- 2 small salmon fillets

- 1 ½ teaspoon salt

- 1 teaspoon black pepper

- 1 tablespoon olive oil

- 1 cup hollandaise sauce, low-carb

Directions:

1. Season well the salmon fillets. Take a medium saucepan or skillet, add oil. Heat over medium heat.

2. Add salmon fillets and stir-cook until evenly seared and cooked well for 4-5 minutes per side. Add asparagus and stir cook for 4-5 more minutes. Serve warm with hollandaise sauce on top.

CPSIA information can be obtained
at www.ICGtesting.com
Printed in the USA
BVHW011154160321
602550BV00024B/540

9 781802 223811